SUGAR DETOX FOR BEGINNERS

A complete guide, recipes and tips to reduce weight naturally and help insulin resistance

Shane Ramiro

Table of contents

Introduction

In the bustling city of Sweetville, where sugar-coated delights beckon from every corner, lived Shane, a young woman with a penchant for sugary indulgence. Cakes, candies, and cookies were her daily companions, and her sweet tooth ruled supreme. However, one day, a wake-up call echoed through her life – a subtle whisper from her tightening jeans and a concerned glance from her reflection in the mirror.

Driven by a desire for change, Shane embarked on a journey that would transform her relationship with sugar. As she navigated the labyrinth of nutrition, battling cravings and resisting the allure of the dessert aisle, Shane discovered the secrets of a sugar-free existence. This led her to compile a comprehensive guide, "Sugar Detox For Beginners," a roadmap for those yearning to break free from the sticky clutches of refined sugars.

Join Shane as she shares her insights, offering practical tips, mouth-watering recipes, and unwavering support for anyone ready to embrace a healthier lifestyle. In Sweetville, where sugar once reigned supreme, a revolution was brewing, and Shane was leading the charge towards a sweeter life without the sugar rush.

Chapter one

Sugar consumption

In the modern world, sugar consumption has become a pervasive aspect of daily life, embedded in our diets through a multitude of processed foods and beverages. While the sweet taste of sugar can be delightful, excessive consumption poses significant health risks. High intake of added sugars is linked to various health issues, including obesity, type 2 diabetes, heart diseases, and dental problems.

Hidden sugars lurk in seemingly innocent products, from sodas and cereals to sauces and dressings. The World Health Organization recommends limiting added sugar intake to less than 10% of total daily calories, emphasizing the importance of mindful choices. Understanding food labels is crucial for identifying sources of hidden sugars and making informed decisions.

Reducing sugar consumption requires a holistic approach, incorporating education, awareness, and behavioral changes. Embracing whole, unprocessed foods, and opting for natural sweeteners can contribute to a healthier lifestyle. Moreover, fostering a conscious relationship with sugar involves mindful eating practices and recognizing the impact of excessive sugar on overall well-being.

As individuals and societies grapple with rising health concerns, addressing and moderating sugar consumption stands as a pivotal step towards cultivating a balanced and sustainable approach to nutrition.

The biomedical impact of sugar in human physiology

The biomedical impact of sugar on human physiology extends beyond the realm of taste and indulgence, influencing various physiological processes with both short-term and long-term consequences. When consumed in excess, refined sugars, such as sucrose and high-fructose corn syrup, can contribute to a range of health issues.

One of the immediate effects of sugar consumption is its impact on blood glucose levels. Rapid spikes in blood sugar trigger the release of insulin, a hormone tasked with regulating glucose. Over time, consistent high sugar intake may lead to insulin resistance, a key factor in the development of type 2 diabetes.

Moreover, excessive sugar consumption is linked to obesity, as sugary foods often contribute to an overconsumption of calories. Adipose tissue, or fat cells, can release inflammatory substances, fostering a pro-inflammatory environment in the body. This chronic inflammation is associated with various metabolic disorders and an increased risk of cardiovascular diseases.

Beyond metabolic concerns, sugar's influence extends to liver health. Excess fructose, in particular, can burden the liver, potentially leading to non-alcoholic fatty liver disease (NAFLD), a condition on the rise globally.

Additionally, sugar plays a role in the complex interplay of neurotransmitters in the brain. While it can provide momentary pleasure by triggering the release of dopamine, chronic overconsumption may lead to desensitization of the brain's reward system, contributing to cravings and addiction-like behaviors.

In summary, the biomedical impact of sugar on human physiology underscores the importance of moderation. Understanding its effects on blood sugar regulation, metabolism, inflammation, and neurological processes is crucial for promoting overall health and preventing the onset of various chronic conditions.

Neurological Impact

Sugar detox involves reducing or eliminating added sugars from the diet, and it can have neurological impacts during the adjustment period. As the body adapts to lower sugar intake, individuals may experience withdrawal-like symptoms, including headaches, irritability, and mood swings. These symptoms are thought to be linked to changes in neurotransmitter levels and the brain's dependence on sugar for energy.

Reducing sugar intake can also positively influence neuroplasticity, the brain's ability to adapt and reorganize itself. Over time, a lower-sugar diet may support improved cognitive function and mood stability. The impact of sugar detox on neurological health varies among individuals, with factors such as overall diet, genetics, and lifestyle playing crucial roles.

It's essential to approach sugar detox gradually, allowing the body and brain to adjust. Staying hydrated, getting adequate sleep, and incorporating nutrient-rich foods can help support the neurological aspects of a sugar detox.

Endocrinological Perspectives

Sugar detox from an endocrinological perspective involves reducing the intake of added sugars to improve hormonal balance, particularly focusing on insulin regulation. High sugar consumption can lead to insulin resistance, where cells become less responsive to insulin, a hormone crucial for glucose uptake.

As individuals undergo a sugar detox, insulin sensitivity tends to improve. This positively influences the endocrine system by helping regulate blood sugar levels more effectively. Lowering sugar intake also contributes to better insulin secretion and reduces the risk of developing insulin resistance, which is associated with various metabolic disorders, including type 2 diabetes.

In addition to insulin, a sugar detox can impact other hormones involved in metabolism. Lowering sugar intake may promote better balance in hormones like leptin and ghrelin, which play roles in hunger and satiety, contributing to improved weight management.

Overall, a sugar detox supports endocrine health by promoting insulin sensitivity and optimizing the hormonal environment related to metabolism and energy balance.

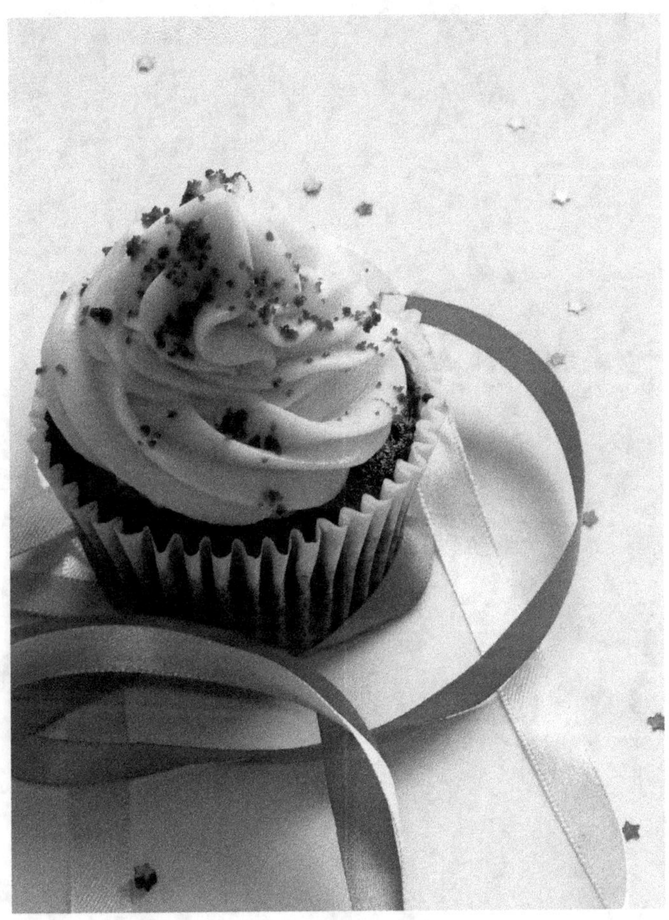

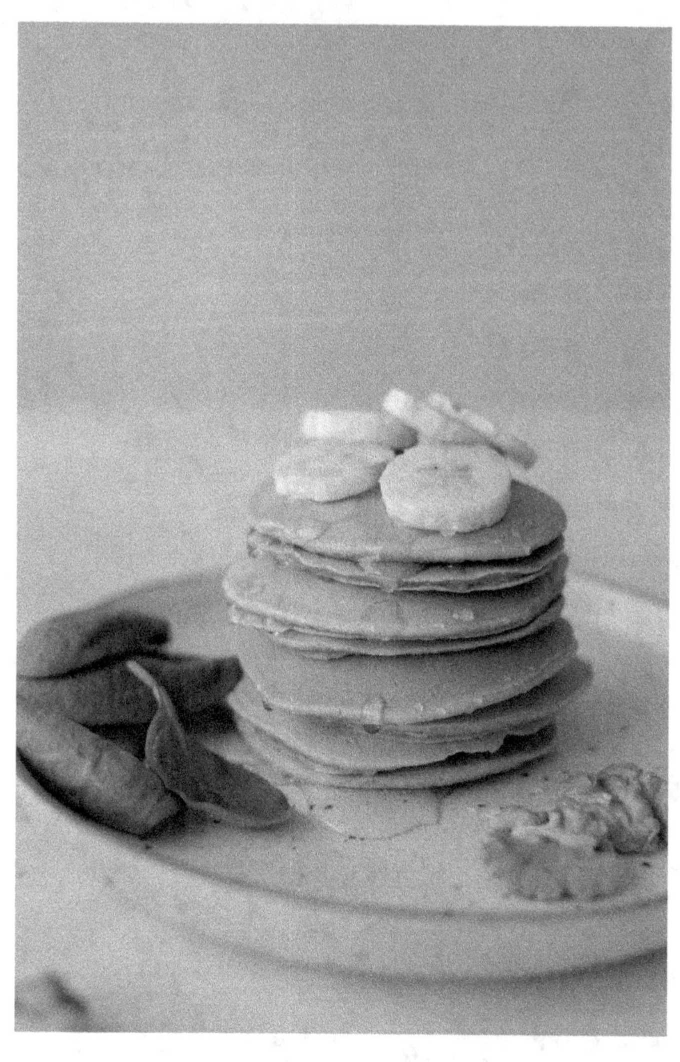

Chapter two

The Rationale for Sugar Detoxification

The rationale for sugar detoxification lies in the numerous health benefits associated with reducing or eliminating added sugars from the diet. Here are key reasons supporting the need for sugar detox:

Metabolic Health: Excessive sugar intake is linked to insulin resistance, a condition where cells become less responsive to insulin. Improving insulin sensitivity through sugar detoxification supports better blood sugar regulation, reducing the risk of metabolic disorders like type 2 diabetes.

Weight Management: High sugar consumption is often associated with weight gain. Sugar detox can contribute to weight loss by reducing calorie intake and preventing the spikes and crashes in blood sugar that can lead to overeating.

Cardiovascular Health: Lowering sugar intake is linked to improvements in various cardiovascular risk factors, including blood pressure and cholesterol levels. Thus, the chance of developing heart disease is decreased.

Brain Health: Excessive sugar consumption has been associated with cognitive decline, mood disorders, and an increased risk of neurodegenerative diseases. Sugar detox may support better cognitive function and mental well-being.

Energy Levels: Relying on sugary foods for energy often leads to energy spikes followed by crashes. A sugar detox promotes stable blood sugar levels, providing sustained energy throughout the day.

Inflammation Reduction: High sugar intake can contribute to chronic inflammation, which is linked to various health issues, including arthritis and heart disease. Sugar detox may help reduce inflammation markers in the body.

Dental Health: Sugars cause cavities and tooth decay. By reducing sugar intake, individuals can promote better oral health.

Improved Hormonal Balance: Lowering sugar intake supports better hormonal regulation, especially insulin, leptin, and ghrelin, which play crucial roles in metabolism and appetite control.

In summary, sugar detoxification is grounded in the potential to enhance overall health by addressing multiple facets of physical well-being, from metabolic function to cardiovascular health and beyond.

Diabetes and Insulin Resistance

Diabetes is a metabolic disorder characterized by elevated blood sugar levels due to inadequate insulin production or impaired insulin function. Insulin, produced by the pancreas, helps regulate blood glucose levels by facilitating the uptake of sugar into cells. Insulin resistance is a key feature of type 2 diabetes, where cells become less responsive to insulin, leading to increased blood sugar levels. Factors contributing to insulin resistance include genetics, obesity, sedentary lifestyle, and certain medical conditions.

Changes in lifestyle are necessary to manage diabetes, including a balanced diet, consistent exercise, and, in some situations, medication. Insulin therapy may be required for those with insufficient insulin production. Early detection and proactive management are crucial in preventing complications like heart disease, kidney damage, and nerve issues associated with diabetes.

Cardiovascular disease

Cardiovascular disease (CVD) refers to a class of disorders that affect the heart and blood vessels, encompassing conditions like coronary artery disease, heart failure, and stroke. Major risk factors include high blood pressure, cholesterol levels, smoking, diabetes, and an unhealthy lifestyle.

Coronary artery disease occurs when blood vessels supplying the heart muscle become narrowed or blocked, leading to chest pain or heart attacks. Heart failure results from the heart's inability to pump blood effectively, while stroke occurs when blood flow to the brain is interrupted.

Preventive measures include adopting a heart-healthy diet, regular exercise, maintaining a healthy weight, and avoiding tobacco. Medications to control blood pressure and cholesterol, as well as surgical interventions, may be recommended based on the severity of the condition.

Awareness, early detection, and lifestyle modifications are crucial in reducing the burden of cardiovascular disease and improving overall heart health. Regular check-ups and adherence to prescribed treatments play a vital role in managing and preventing cardiovascular issues.

Obesity and related complications

Obesity is a medical condition characterized by excessive body weight due to an accumulation of fat. It is a complex issue influenced by genetics, environment, and lifestyle choices. Complications from obesity include the following:

1. Type 2 Diabetes: Obesity is a significant risk factor for insulin resistance and type 2 diabetes. Excess fat can impair insulin function, leading to elevated blood sugar levels.

2. Cardiovascular Disease: Obesity increases the risk of heart disease and stroke by contributing to conditions like high blood pressure, high cholesterol levels, and atherosclerosis.

3. Joint Problems: Excessive weight puts added stress on joints, leading to conditions like osteoarthritis, particularly in weight-bearing joints like the knees and hips.

4. Respiratory Issues: Obesity can cause or worsen respiratory problems, including sleep apnea, asthma, and shortness of breath.

5. Liver Disease: Non-alcoholic fatty liver disease (NAFLD) is common in obese individuals, potentially progressing to more severe conditions like liver cirrhosis.

6. Cancer: Obesity is associated with an increased risk of certain cancers, including breast, colorectal, and prostate cancer.

7. Psychological Impact: Obesity can contribute to mental health issues such as depression, low self-esteem, and body image concerns.

Addressing obesity involves a holistic approach, including lifestyle changes such as a balanced diet and regular physical activity. Medical interventions, like medications or surgery, may be considered in severe cases.

Early intervention and sustained efforts are crucial in preventing and managing obesity-related complications.

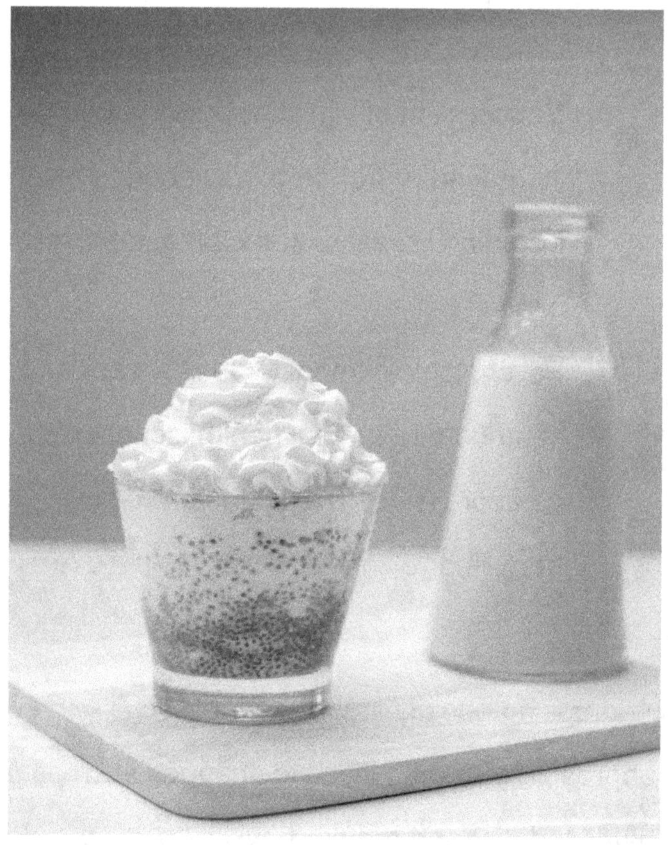

Chapter three

Physiological aspect of sugar consumption

Sugar consumption has various physiological effects on the body, influencing multiple systems:

1. **Blood Sugar Levels:** Consuming sugar leads to a rapid increase in blood glucose levels. This prompts the pancreas to release insulin to help cells absorb and use the sugar for energy.

2. **Insulin Response:** Over time, excessive sugar intake can contribute to insulin resistance, where cells become less responsive to insulin. This condition

is linked to the development of type 2 diabetes.

3. **Weight Gain:** High sugar intake, especially in the form of added sugars and sugary beverages, can contribute to weight gain. The excess calories from sugar are often stored as fat.

4. **Inflammation:** Chronic consumption of sugar may lead to increased inflammation in the body, which is associated with various health issues, including cardiovascular disease and other chronic conditions.

5. **Liver Function:** The liver plays a crucial role in processing sugar. Excessive sugar intake, particularly fructose, can lead to non-alcoholic fatty liver disease (NAFLD) and may contribute to liver dysfunction.

6. **Hormonal Impact:** Sugar consumption can influence hormones related to hunger and satiety, potentially leading to overeating and disrupted appetite regulation.

7. **Dental Health:** High sugar intake is a major contributor to tooth decay. Sugar is the food source for oral bacteria, which produce acids that damage tooth enamel.

8. **Brain Function:** Some studies suggest a link between high sugar intake and impaired cognitive function. Excessive sugar consumption may contribute to issues like poor memory and decreased attention span.

Moderating sugar intake, especially added sugars, is important for maintaining overall health. Choosing whole, unprocessed foods and being mindful of hidden sugars in packaged products can help mitigate the potential negative physiological effects of excessive sugar consumption.

Sugar and Mood Fluctuations

Consuming sugary foods can lead to mood fluctuations due to various physiological and psychological factors:

1. Blood Sugar Spikes and Crashes: Rapid spikes in blood sugar levels after consuming sugary foods are often followed by crashes. These fluctuations can lead to mood swings, irritability, and fatigue.

2. Insulin Response: The body releases
    insulin to help regulate blood sugar
    levels after consuming sugar. The
    subsequent drop in blood sugar levels
    may contribute to feelings of irritability
    and low energy.

3. Serotonin Levels: Sugar intake can
    influence serotonin, a neurotransmitter
    associated with mood regulation. While
    sugar initially increases serotonin levels,
    the subsequent drop may affect mood,
    potentially contributing to feelings of
    sadness or irritability.

4. Brain Fog: Excessive sugar
    consumption has been linked to
    cognitive issues, including difficulty
    concentrating and mental fog. These
    factors can impact overall mood and
    productivity.

5. Addiction-like Response: Sugar
    activates reward centers in the brain,
    leading to a temporary feeling of
    pleasure. However, the subsequent
    withdrawal or "craving" phase can
    contribute to mood swings and cravings
    for more sugary foods.
6. Inflammation: Chronic consumption of
    sugary foods may contribute to
    inflammation, which has been linked to
    mood disorders such as depression.
    The inflammatory response could
    influence neurotransmitter function and
    mood regulation.

While the impact of sugar on mood can vary
among individuals, maintaining a balanced diet
with moderate sugar intake is generally
advisable for overall mental and emotional

well-being. Choosing complex carbohydrates, such as whole grains and fruits, over refined sugars can help mitigate mood fluctuations associated with rapid blood sugar changes.

Sugar and Cognitive Decline

Excessive sugar intake has been associated with cognitive decline and an increased risk of conditions like dementia and Alzheimer's disease. Here are some ways in which sugar may contribute to cognitive decline:

1. **Insulin Resistance:** Prolonged consumption of high levels of sugar can lead to insulin resistance, impairing the brain's ability to use glucose effectively. This insulin resistance has been linked to cognitive dysfunction and an elevated risk of neurodegenerative diseases.

2. **Inflammation:** Chronic consumption of sugary foods may contribute to systemic inflammation, which can negatively impact the brain. Inflammation is considered a potential factor in the development and progression of cognitive decline.

3. **Brain Structure and Function:** Studies suggest that diets high in sugar may affect the structure and function of the hippocampus, a brain region crucial for memory and learning. Changes in the hippocampus are often observed in individuals with cognitive disorders.

4. **Advanced Glycation End Products (AGEs):** The interaction between sugars and proteins can lead to the formation of AGEs, which accumulate in the brain over time. High levels of AGEs have

been associated with oxidative stress and inflammation, contributing to cognitive impairment.

5. **Blood Vessel Health:** Excessive sugar consumption can contribute to vascular issues, affecting blood vessel health. Impaired blood flow to the brain is a risk factor for cognitive decline and dementia.

6. **Neurotransmitter Imbalance:** Sugar intake can influence neurotransmitter levels, impacting mood and cognitive function. Fluctuations in neurotransmitters may contribute to cognitive issues, including memory and attention deficits.

Adopting a balanced diet that limits added sugars and focuses on whole, nutrient-dense foods is crucial for maintaining brain health. Additionally, staying physically active, managing stress, and maintaining a healthy lifestyle contribute to overall cognitive well-being and may help reduce the risk of cognitive decline associated with excessive sugar consumption.

Gender Specific Consideration in Sugar Detoxification

While sugar detoxification principles generally apply to all individuals, there can be gender-specific considerations due to variations in metabolism, hormonal differences, and nutritional needs. Here are some considerations for sugar detoxification based on gender:

1. **Hormonal Influence:**

- Females: Hormonal fluctuations during the menstrual cycle may affect cravings. Strategies to manage sugar detox may need to account for these fluctuations, especially during the premenstrual phase when some women may experience increased cravings.
- Males: Hormonal differences in males might influence how the body processes sugar, potentially affecting detox outcomes. Individual variations in testosterone levels could play a role in energy metabolism.

2. **Nutritional Needs:**

- Females: Women may have specific nutritional needs, especially during pregnancy or menstruation, that should be considered during sugar detox. It is vital to make sure you are getting enough of the necessary nutrients.
- Males: Men might have different caloric and nutrient requirements. Balancing nutrient intake while reducing sugar can help maintain overall health.

3. **Emotional Aspects:**

- Females: Emotional eating patterns, which can be influenced by hormonal changes, may impact women more significantly. Recognizing and addressing emotional triggers during sugar detox can be crucial.

- Males: Men may also experience emotional connections to food, and addressing stress or emotional eating patterns is important for successful sugar detox.

4. Physical Activity:

- Females: Exercise can play a role in managing hormonal fluctuations and supporting sugar detox. Tailoring exercise routines to menstrual cycles may be beneficial.
- Males: Regular physical activity is essential for both genders during sugar detox, but individual preferences and fitness goals may vary.

5. **Support Systems:**

- Females: Women might benefit from support systems that acknowledge hormonal influences and provide encouragement during challenging periods.
- Males: Men may also find support valuable, particularly if societal expectations around diet and masculinity impact their approach to sugar detox.

In both genders, personalized approaches considering individual health status, lifestyle, and preferences are key. Consulting with healthcare professionals or nutritionists can help tailor sugar detoxification plans to specific gender-related considerations.

Gender Difference in Insulin sensitivity

Gender differences in insulin sensitivity can be influenced by various factors, including hormonal variations, body composition, and distribution of fat. Here are some key considerations:

1. **Hormonal Influence:**

- Females: Hormonal fluctuations throughout the menstrual cycle, particularly during the luteal phase, can impact insulin sensitivity. Insulin sensitivity tends to be lower in the days leading up to menstruation, potentially affecting glucose metabolism.
- Males: Testosterone, more prevalent in males, may contribute to better insulin

sensitivity. However, higher levels of visceral fat, often associated with males, can counteract this positive effect.

2. Body Composition:

- Females: Women generally have a higher percentage of body fat than men, and fat distribution is often subcutaneous. Subcutaneous fat is associated with better insulin sensitivity compared to visceral fat.
- Males: Men tend to accumulate more visceral fat, particularly in the abdominal area. Visceral fat is linked to insulin resistance, potentially offsetting the benefits of higher testosterone levels.

3. Fat Distribution:

- Females: The subcutaneous fat distribution in women, especially in the gluteofemoral region, may have a protective effect on insulin sensitivity. However, changes in fat distribution during menopause can alter this dynamic.
- Males: Central or abdominal obesity in men is associated with a higher risk of insulin resistance. The distribution of fat plays a crucial role in determining overall metabolic health.

4. Physical Activity:

- Females: Regular physical activity can improve insulin sensitivity in both genders, but women may derive additional benefits, especially post-menopause, as exercise helps counteract age-related declines in insulin sensitivity.

- Males: Exercise, particularly resistance training, is associated with improved insulin sensitivity in men. Physical activity helps regulate glucose metabolism and enhances insulin action.

5. **Aging**:

- Females: Insulin sensitivity tends to decrease with age, and menopausal hormonal changes can further impact glucose metabolism in women.

- Males: Aging also affects insulin
  sensitivity in men, but the decline may
  be more gradual compared to women,
  influenced by factors such as
  testosterone levels.

Understanding these gender-specific factors is important in tailoring approaches to manage insulin sensitivity. Both men and women can benefit from a healthy lifestyle, including regular exercise, balanced nutrition, and weight management, to optimize insulin sensitivity and overall metabolic health.

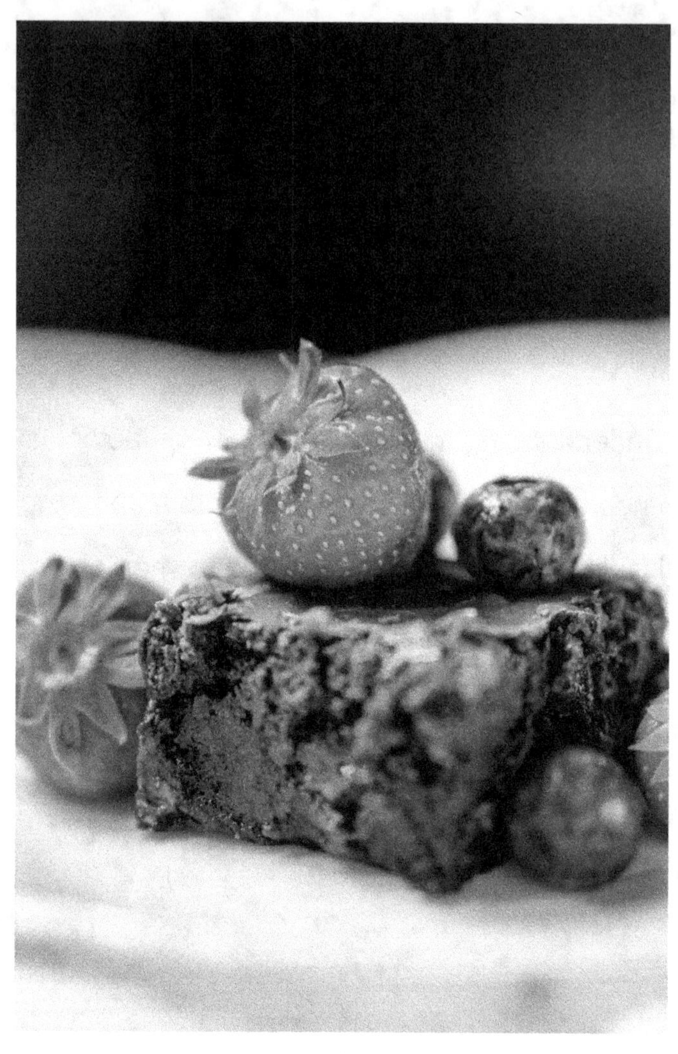

Chapter four

Hormonal interactions with sugar intake

Sugar intake can interact with hormonal regulation in various ways, influencing metabolic processes, appetite, and mood. Here are some key hormonal interactions associated with sugar consumption:

1. **Insulin and Glucagon:**
    - Insulin: Released in response to increased blood sugar levels, insulin facilitates the uptake of glucose into cells for energy or storage. High sugar intake can lead to frequent insulin spikes,

potentially contributing to insulin resistance over time.

- Glucagon: This hormone works in opposition to insulin, promoting the release of glucose from the liver when blood sugar levels drop. Excessive sugar consumption may disrupt the balance between insulin and glucagon.

2. **Leptin and Ghrelin:**

- Leptin: Often referred to as the "satiety hormone," leptin signals to the brain that you're full. Chronic high sugar intake may contribute to leptin resistance, disrupting the body's ability to regulate appetite.

- Ghrelin:Ghrelin: Also referred to as the "hunger hormone," this hormone increases hunger. Sweetener. Sugar consumption can influence ghrelin levels, potentially leading to increased feelings of hunger.

3. **Cortisol:**

   - Cortisol: Released in response to stress, cortisol can influence blood sugar levels. Chronic stress combined with high sugar intake may contribute to elevated cortisol levels, impacting insulin sensitivity and promoting fat storage.

4. **Serotonin:**

   - Serotonin: Sugar can temporarily boost serotonin levels, providing

a mood lift. However, the
subsequent drop in blood sugar
may lead to mood swings and
cravings, potentially contributing
to a cycle of sugar consumption
for mood regulation.

5. **Estrogen and Testosterone:**

   - Estrogen: Hormonal fluctuations,
     such as those during the
     menstrual cycle, can affect how
     the body responds to sugar.
     Changes in estrogen levels may
     influence insulin sensitivity and
     cravings in women.

   - Testosterone: High sugar intake
     may contribute to lower
     testosterone levels, impacting
     muscle mass and potentially

affecting metabolism in both men
and women.

Understanding these hormonal interactions
highlights the intricate relationship between
sugar consumption and the body's regulatory
systems. Chronic exposure to high levels of
sugar, especially added sugars, can disrupt
these hormonal pathways, potentially leading
to metabolic issues, weight gain, and an
increased risk of conditions like insulin
resistance and type 2 diabetes. Adopting a
balanced diet with mindful sugar consumption
is essential for maintaining hormonal balance
and overall health.

A practical Approach of sugar detox recipes

Embarking on a sugar detox involves reducing or eliminating added sugars from your diet. Here's a practical approach with a few recipes to help you navigate a sugar detox:

Breakfast:

1. Quinoa Breakfast Bowl:

- Ingredients: Cooked quinoa, fresh berries, a sprinkle of nuts, and a dash of cinnamon.
- Directions: Mix the ingredients in a bowl for a nutrient-dense, sugar-free breakfast.

2. Veggie Omelette:

- Ingredients: Eggs, diced bell peppers,
  spinach, and tomatoes.
- Directions: Whisk eggs and cook with
  veggies for a satisfying, low-sugar
  breakfast.

Snacks:

3. Greek Yogurt Parfait:

- Ingredients: Plain Greek yogurt,
  unsweetened granola, and sliced
  strawberries.
- Directions: Layer the ingredients for a
  protein-packed, naturally sweetened
  snack.

4. Veggie Sticks with Hummus:

- Ingredients: Carrot, cucumber, and celery sticks with homemade hummus.
- Directions: Dip veggies into hummus for a satisfying and fiber-rich snack.

Lunch:

5. Grilled Chicken Salad:

- Ingredients: Grilled chicken, mixed greens, cherry tomatoes, cucumber, and a vinaigrette dressing.
- Directions: Toss the ingredients for a flavorful, sugar-free lunch option.

6. Quinoa and Black Bean Bowl:

- Ingredients: Cooked quinoa, black beans, diced avocado, and lime juice.

- Directions: Mix the ingredients for a protein-rich, low-sugar lunch.

Dinner:

7. Baked Salmon with Roasted Vegetables:

- Ingredients: Salmon fillet, broccoli, cauliflower, and olive oil.
- Directions: Bake salmon and veggies for a nutritious, sugar-free dinner.

8. Zucchini Noodles with Pesto:

- Ingredients: Spiralized zucchini, homemade basil pesto, and cherry tomatoes.
- Directions: Toss the ingredients for a low-carb, sugar-free pasta alternative.

Dessert:

9. Berry and Coconut Chia Pudding:

- Ingredients: Chia seeds, coconut milk, mixed berries.
- Directions: Mix and refrigerate for a delicious, naturally sweetened dessert.

10. Baked Apples with Cinnamon:

- Ingredients: Sliced apples, cinnamon, and a touch of coconut oil.
- Directions: Bake until tender for a warm, sugar-free treat.

Beverages:

11. Infused Water:

- Ingredients: Water with cucumber slices, mint, and lemon.
- Directions: Let it infuse for a refreshing, sugar-free drink.

12. Herbal Tea:

- Ingredients: Choose unsweetened herbal teas for a calming, sugar-free option.

Remember to read labels and opt for whole, unprocessed foods during your sugar detox. Gradually reintroduce natural sugars from fruits and monitor how your body responds. Staying hydrated and incorporating a variety of nutrient-dense foods will support your journey towards a reduced-sugar lifestyle.

Breakfast Options

Certainly! Here are some balanced and nutritious breakfast options:

1. Overnight Oats:

- Ingredients: Rolled oats, milk or plant-based alternative, Greek yogurt, fruits, nuts, and a drizzle of honey.
- Preparation: Mix ingredients in a jar, refrigerate overnight, and grab a ready-to-eat breakfast in the morning.

2. Avocado Toast:

- Ingredients: Whole-grain toast, mashed avocado, cherry tomatoes, a sprinkle of feta cheese, and a dash of olive oil.

- Preparation: Spread mashed avocado
  on toast and top with sliced tomatoes,
  feta, and olive oil.

3. Greek Yogurt Parfait:

- Greek yogurt, granola, mixed berries,
  and honey drizzled over are the
  ingredients.
- Preparation: Layer yogurt, granola, and
  berries in a glass or bowl for a tasty and
  protein-rich breakfast.

4. Smoothie Bowl:

- Ingredients: Blended frozen fruits
  (berries, banana), spinach, Greek
  yogurt, and a sprinkle of chia seeds.

- Preparation: Blend ingredients and top with chia seeds for added texture and nutrients.

5. Egg and Veggie Wrap:

- Ingredients: Whole-grain wrap, scrambled eggs, sautéed vegetables (bell peppers, spinach), and a sprinkle of cheese.
- Preparation: Fill the wrap with scrambled eggs, veggies, and cheese, then fold it into a wrap.

6. Chia Seed Pudding:

- Ingredients: Chia seeds, almond milk, vanilla extract, and fresh fruit.

- Preparation: Mix chia seeds with almond milk and vanilla, refrigerate until it thickens, then top with fresh fruit.

7. Peanut Butter Banana Toast:

- Ingredients: Whole-grain toast, peanut butter, banana slices, and a sprinkle of cinnamon.
- Preparation: Spread peanut butter on toast and add banana slices, finishing with a dash of cinnamon.

8. Breakfast Burrito:

- Ingredients: Whole-grain tortilla, scrambled eggs, black beans, salsa, and avocado.

- Preparation: Fill the tortilla with scrambled eggs, black beans, salsa, and sliced avocado, then fold into a burrito.

9. Quinoa Breakfast Bowl:

- Ingredients: Cooked quinoa, mixed berries, chopped nuts, and a dollop of Greek yogurt.
- Preparation: Combine cooked quinoa with berries, nuts, and Greek yogurt for a protein-packed breakfast.

10. Cottage Cheese with Pineapple:

- Ingredients: Cottage cheese and fresh pineapple chunks.

- Preparation: Mix cottage cheese with pineapple chunks for a quick and protein-rich breakfast.

These options offer a mix of carbohydrates, protein, healthy fats, and fiber, providing sustained energy to kickstart your day. Adjust portion sizes based on your individual nutritional needs.

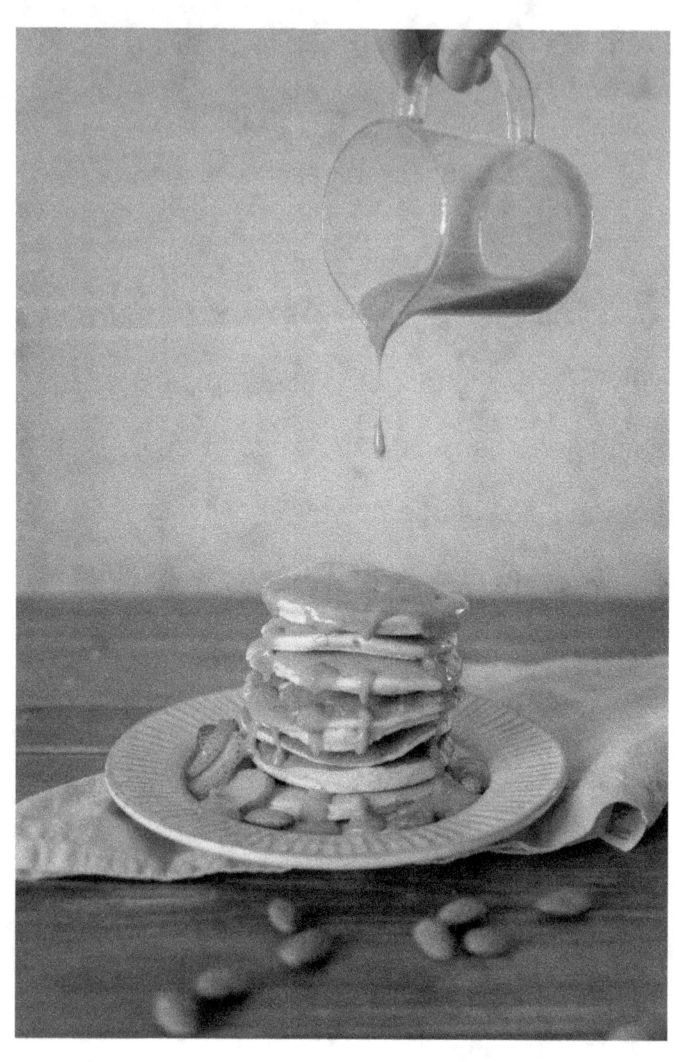

Chapter five

Nutritional balancing for sustained energy

Balancing your nutritional intake is crucial for sustained energy throughout the day. Here's a guide to achieving nutritional balance:

**1. Complex Carbohydrates:

- Sources: Whole grains (quinoa, brown rice), legumes, vegetables.
- Why: Provide a steady release of glucose for sustained energy.

**2. Protein:

- Sources: Lean meats, fish, poultry, tofu, legumes, eggs, dairy.

- Why: Supports muscle health, helps control appetite, and provides lasting energy.

3. Healthy Fats:

- Sources: Avocado, nuts, seeds, olive oil, fatty fish.
- Why: Essential for brain function and satiety, helps regulate blood sugar.

4. Fruits and Vegetables:

- Sources: A rainbow of vibrant fruits and veggies
- Why: Rich in vitamins, minerals, and antioxidants for overall health and sustained energy.

5. **Hydration:

- Sources: Water, herbal teas.

- Why: Dehydration can lead to fatigue; adequate hydration supports bodily functions.

6. **Regular Meals and Snacks:

- Timing: Spread meals evenly throughout the day, include healthy snacks.

- Why: Maintains a consistent energy supply and prevents blood sugar fluctuations.

7. **Fiber:

- Sources: Whole grains, fruits, vegetables, legumes.

- Why: Supports digestion, helps stabilize blood sugar, and provides lasting energy.

8. Micronutrients:

- Sources: Include a variety of foods for a broad range of vitamins and minerals.
- Why: Essential for overall health, energy production, and immune function.

9. Limit Added Sugars:

- Sources: Minimize sugary snacks, sodas, and processed foods.
- Why: Prevents energy crashes and supports stable blood sugar levels.

10. Caffeine Moderation:

- Sources: Tea, coffee (in moderation).

- Why: Can enhance alertness, but excessive intake can lead to energy crashes.

**11. Balanced Meals:

- Components: Include a combination of carbohydrates, protein, and healthy fats in each meal.
- Why: Optimizes nutrient absorption and provides sustained energy.

**12. Mindful Eating:

- Practice: Eat slowly, pay attention to hunger and fullness cues.
- Why: Enhances digestion and allows for better nutrient absorption.

13. Whole Foods:

- Preference: Choose whole, unprocessed foods over highly processed options.
- Why: Whole foods provide a broader range of nutrients and support overall health.

14. Sleep:

- Prioritize: Aim for 7-9 hours of quality sleep each night.
- Why: Essential for energy restoration and overall well-being.

15. Physical Activity:

- Frequent Exercise: Incorporate both strength and aerobic workouts.

- Why: Enhances overall energy levels and supports metabolic health.

Adopting these nutritional practices as part of a balanced lifestyle can help you maintain sustained energy levels throughout the day. Remember that individual needs may vary, and consulting with a healthcare professional or registered dietitian for personalized advice is always beneficial.

Lunch and Dinner Ideas

Certainly! Here are some delicious and nutritious lunch and dinner ideas:

Lunch:

1. Grilled Chicken Salad:

- Ingredients: Grilled chicken breast, mixed greens, cherry tomatoes, cucumber, feta cheese, and balsamic vinaigrette.
- Preparation: Toss all ingredients together for a light and satisfying salad.

2. Quinoa and Black Bean Bowl:

- Ingredients: Cooked quinoa, black beans, corn, avocado, cherry tomatoes, and lime dressing.
- Preparation: Mix the ingredients and drizzle with lime dressing for a flavorful and protein-packed bowl.

3. Mediterranean Chickpea Wrap:

- Ingredients: Whole-grain wrap, hummus, chickpeas, cherry

tomatoes, cucumber, red onion,
and feta cheese.

- Preparation: Assemble the wrap
  with hummus, chickpeas,
  veggies, and feta.

4. Salmon and Avocado Wrap:

   - Ingredients: Whole-grain wrap,
     grilled salmon, avocado slices,
     lettuce, and a yogurt-dill sauce.

   - Preparation: Fill the wrap with
     grilled salmon, avocado, lettuce,
     and drizzle with yogurt-dill sauce.

5. Vegetarian Quinoa Stir-Fry:

   - Ingredients: Quinoa, tofu or
     chickpeas, colorful stir-fried
     vegetables, and soy-ginger
     sauce.

   - Preparation: Stir-fry tofu or
     chickpeas with veggies and

quinoa, then toss with soy-ginger sauce.

Dinner:

1. Baked Chicken with Sweet Potato and Broccoli:
   - Ingredients: Baked chicken breast, roasted sweet potatoes, and steamed broccoli.
   - Preparation: Bake chicken, roast sweet potatoes, and steam broccoli for a simple and nutritious dinner.
2. Vegetarian Lentil Soup:
   - Ingredients: Lentils, carrots, celery, tomatoes, spinach, vegetable broth, and spices.
   - Preparation: Simmer lentils and veggies in vegetable broth with

spices for a hearty and
comforting soup.

3. Shrimp and Quinoa Stir-Fry:

    o   Ingredients: Shrimp, quinoa,
        stir-fried bell peppers, snap peas,
        and a sesame-soy sauce.

    o   Preparation: Stir-fry shrimp and
        veggies, mix with quinoa, and
        drizzle with sesame-soy sauce.

4. Eggplant and Chickpea Curry:

    o   Ingredients: Eggplant, chickpeas,
        tomatoes, coconut milk, and curry
        spices.

    o   Preparation: Cook eggplant,
        chickpeas, and tomatoes in a
        coconut milk curry sauce for a
        flavorful vegetarian curry.

5. Grilled Veggie and Chicken Kabobs:

- Ingredients: Grilled chicken skewers with bell peppers, cherry tomatoes, zucchini, and mushrooms.
- Preparation: Thread chicken and veggies onto skewers, grill until cooked, and serve with a side of whole grain.

Vegetarians and vegans alternative

Absolutely! Here are some delicious vegetarian and vegan alternatives for both lunch and dinner:

Vegetarian Lunch:

1. Caprese Salad Wrap:

- o Ingredients: Whole-grain wrap, fresh mozzarella, tomato slices, basil leaves, and balsamic glaze.
  - o Preparation: Assemble the wrap with mozzarella, tomatoes, and basil, drizzle with balsamic glaze.

2. Chickpea Salad Sandwich:
  - o Ingredients: Mashed chickpeas, celery, red onion, vegan mayo, mustard, and whole-grain bread.
  - o Preparation: Mix mashed chickpeas with veggies and spread on whole-grain bread for a tasty sandwich.

3. Spinach and Feta Stuffed Portobello Mushrooms:
  - o Ingredients: Portobello mushrooms, spinach, feta

cheese, garlic, and cherry
tomatoes.

- o Preparation: Stuff mushrooms
  with a mixture of sautéed
  spinach, garlic, feta, and
  tomatoes, then bake until tender.

4. Sweet Potato and Black Bean
Quesadilla:

- o Ingredients: Whole-grain tortilla,
  sweet potato mash, black beans,
  corn, avocado, and vegan
  cheese.
- o Preparation: Assemble the
  quesadilla with sweet potato,
  beans, corn, avocado, and vegan
  cheese, then grill until crispy.

5. Mediterranean Quinoa Salad:

- o Ingredients: Quinoa, cherry
  tomatoes, cucumber, olives, red

onion, and a lemon-tahini
dressing.

- ○ Preparation: Toss cooked quinoa
  with veggies and drizzle with a
  lemon-tahini dressing for a
  refreshing salad.

Vegan Dinner:

1. Vegan Lentil Bolognese:
   - ○ Ingredients: Lentils, crushed
     tomatoes, onion, garlic, carrots,
     and whole-grain pasta.
   - ○ Preparation: Cook lentils with
     veggies and tomatoes, then
     serve over whole-grain pasta.
2. Black beans and Quinoa Stuffed Bell
   Peppers:

- Ingredients: Bell peppers, quinoa, black beans, corn, salsa, and avocado.
- Preparation: Stuff bell peppers with a mixture of quinoa, black beans, corn, and top with salsa and avocado.

3. Vegan Chickpea Curry:
   - Ingredients: Chickpeas, coconut milk, tomatoes, spinach, and curry spices.
   - Preparation: Simmer chickpeas and veggies in coconut milk with curry spices for a flavorful vegan curry.

4. Cauliflower and Chickpea Buddha Bowl:
   - Ingredients: Roasted cauliflower, chickpeas, quinoa, avocado, and a tahini dressing.

- Preparation: Arrange roasted cauliflower, chickpeas, and avocado over quinoa, then drizzle with tahini dressing.

5. Vegan Stir-Fried Tofu and Vegetables:
   - Ingredients: Tofu, broccoli, bell peppers, snow peas, and a soy-ginger sauce.
   - Preparation: Stir-fry tofu and veggies with a soy-ginger sauce and serve over brown rice.

These vegetarian and vegan options are rich in plant-based proteins, fiber, and nutrients, providing a variety of flavors and textures for a satisfying and well-rounded meal. Adjust recipes based on personal preferences and dietary needs.

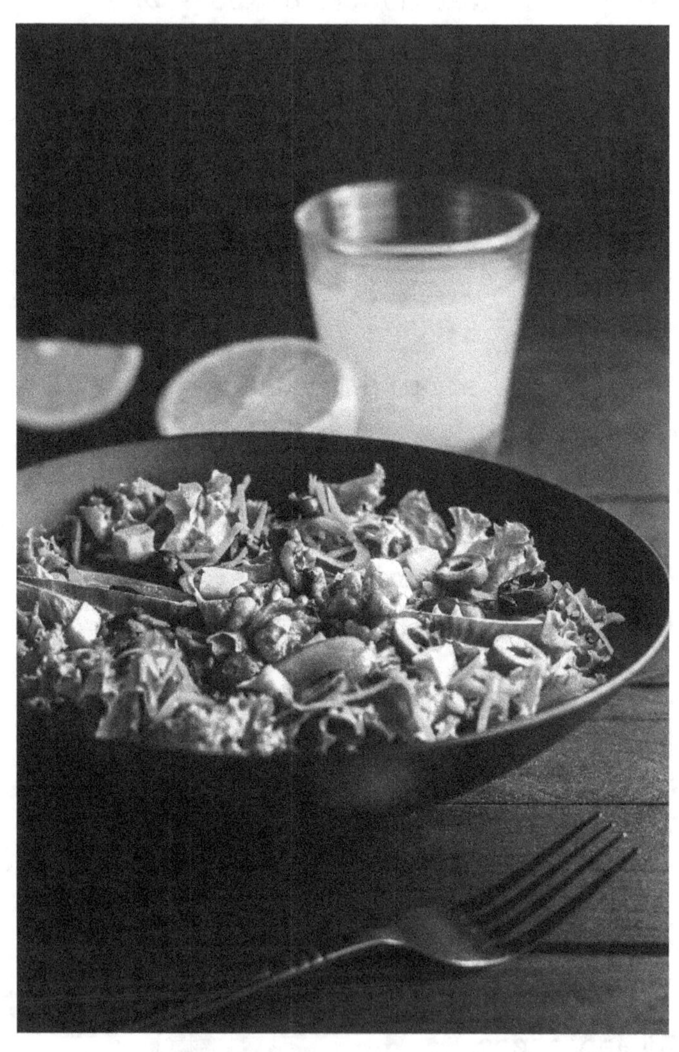

Chapter six

Snacks and Beverages

Certainly! Here are some healthy and tasty snack ideas, along with refreshing beverage options:

Snacks:

1. Homemade Trail Mix:
    - Ingredients: Mixed nuts, seeds, dried fruit, and dark chocolate.
    - Preparation: Mix your favorite nuts, seeds, and dried fruits for a custom trail mix.
2. Veggies and Hummus:
    - Ingredients: Sliced carrots, cucumber, bell peppers, and hummus.

- Preparation: Dip veggies in hummus for a satisfying and nutritious snack.

3. Apple Slices with Almond Butter:

   - Ingredients: Apple slices and almond butter.

   - Preparation: Spread almond butter on apple slices for a sweet and crunchy combo.

4. Greek Yogurt with Berries:

   - Ingredients: Plain Greek yogurt and mixed berries.

   - Preparation: Top Greek yogurt with fresh or frozen berries for a protein-packed snack.

5. Roasted Chickpeas:

   - Ingredients: Chickpeas, olive oil, and spices (like cumin or paprika).

○ Preparation: Roast chickpeas in the oven until crispy for a crunchy and fiber-rich snack.

6. Whole Grain Crackers with Avocado:

   ○ Ingredients: Whole grain crackers and sliced avocado.

   ○ Preparation: Top crackers with avocado slices for a satisfying and heart-healthy snack.

Beverages:

1. Infused Water:

   ○ Ingredients: Water with cucumber slices, mint, and lemon.

   ○ Preparation: Let it infuse for a refreshing, sugar-free drink.

2. Herbal Tea:

- Ingredients: Choose
    unsweetened herbal teas for a
    calming, sugar-free option.

3. Green Smoothie:

    - Ingredients: Spinach, banana,
    pineapple, almond milk, and chia
    seeds.

    - Preparation: Blend ingredients for
    a nutrient-packed and hydrating
    smoothie.

4. Iced Peppermint Tea:

    - Ingredients: Peppermint tea
    bags, ice, and a splash of lemon.

    - Preparation: Brew peppermint
    tea, let it cool, add ice, and a
    squeeze of lemon for a refreshing
    beverage.

5. Coconut Water:

- o Ingredients: Unsweetened
    coconut water.
  - o Preparation: Enjoy coconut water
    on its own for a natural and
    hydrating drink.
6. Vegetable Juice:
  - o Ingredients: Tomatoes, celery,
    carrots, and a dash of hot sauce.
  - o Preparation: Juice vegetables for
    a savory and nutrient-packed
    beverage.

These snack and beverage options offer a mix
of flavors, textures, and nutritional benefits.
Whether you're looking for something crunchy,
sweet, or hydrating, these ideas can keep you
satisfied throughout the day. Adjust portion
sizes based on your preferences and dietary
needs.

Strategies for sugar-free snacking

Opting for sugar-free snacks involves choosing options that are low in added sugars while still being satisfying and enjoyable. Here are some strategies for sugar-free snacking:

1. Choose Whole Fruits:

- Enjoy whole fruits like apples, berries, or oranges. They provide fiber, vital minerals, and a naturally pleasant taste.

2. Incorporate Nuts and Seeds:

- Snack on a handful of nuts (almonds, walnuts, or pistachios) or seeds (sunflower seeds, pumpkin seeds). They offer a satisfying crunch and are rich in healthy fats.

3. Greek Yogurt with Berries:

- Opt for plain Greek yogurt and add fresh berries for sweetness. Greek yogurt is high in protein, keeping you full for longer.

4. Veggie Sticks with Hummus:

- Dip colorful vegetable sticks—such as bell peppers, cucumbers, and carrots—into hummus. Hummus provides a tasty and protein-rich option.

5. Cheese and Whole Grain Crackers:

- Pair a small serving of cheese with whole grain crackers for a balanced and satisfying snack.

6. Hard-Boiled Eggs:

- Hard-boiled eggs are a protein-rich option that can help curb hunger and provide essential nutrients.

7. Nut Butter on Rice Cakes:

- Spread natural nut butter (like almond or peanut butter) on whole grain rice cakes for a tasty and filling snack.

8. Avocado on Whole Grain Toast:

- Mash avocado and spread it on whole grain toast. This combination offers healthy fats and fiber.

9. Trail Mix with Nuts and Seeds:

- Make your own trail mix with a mix of unsalted nuts, seeds, and a small amount of dried fruits.

10. Cottage Cheese with Pineapple:

- Cottage cheese paired with fresh pineapple chunks is a delicious and satisfying option.

11. Veggie Salsa with Whole Grain Pita:

- Create a veggie salsa with tomatoes, onions, and cilantro. Pair it with whole grain pita for a flavorful snack.

12. Popcorn with Olive Oil and Herbs:

- Air-popped popcorn drizzled with a bit of olive oil and your favorite herbs is a light and crunchy option.

13. Seaweed Snacks:

- Crispy seaweed snacks are low in calories and offer a unique texture. They come in a variety of tastes.

14. Edamame:

- Steamed edamame sprinkled with a bit of sea salt is a protein-rich and satisfying snack.

15. Yogurt Parfait with Nuts:

* Layer plain yogurt with nuts, seeds, and a small amount of natural sweeteners like honey or maple syrup.

16. Sugar-Free Nut Bars:

* Look for nut bars that are free from added sugars or make your own by combining nuts, seeds, and a natural sweetener like dates.

17. Vegetable Chips:

* Bake your own veggie chips using zucchini, sweet potatoes, or kale for a crunchy and nutritious snack.

When choosing sugar-free snacks, it's essential to read labels, opt for whole, unprocessed foods, and be mindful of portion sizes. These strategies can help you enjoy satisfying snacks while minimizing added sugars in your diet.

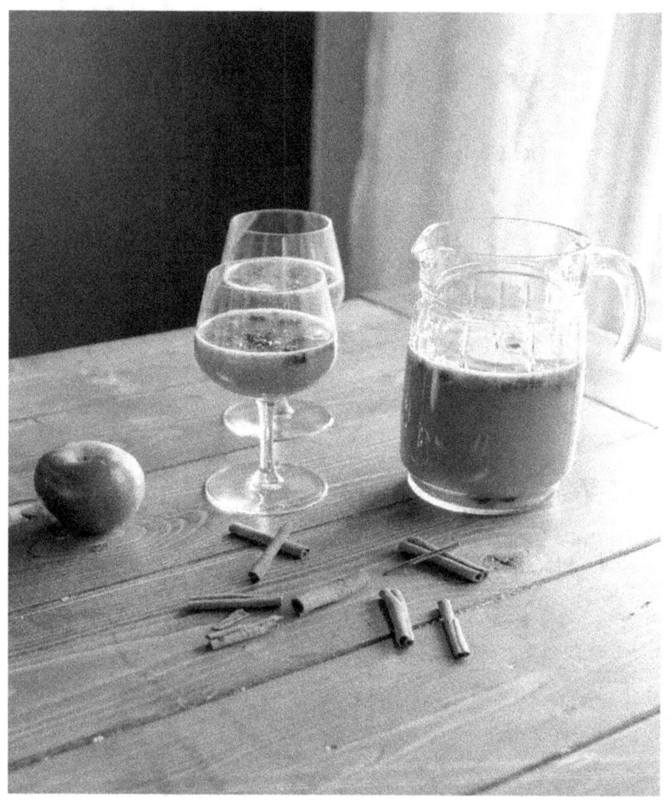

Chapter seven

Replacing sugary beverages with healthful choices

Replacing sugary beverages with healthier alternatives is a positive step towards improving your overall health. Here are some healthful choices to consider:

1. Water:

- Why: Staying hydrated is crucial for overall health. Water is calorie-free, essential for bodily functions, and helps with digestion.

2. Herbal Tea:

- Why: Herbal teas come in various flavors and are caffeine-free. They can be enjoyed hot or cold, providing

hydration without added sugars.

3. Infused Water:

- Why: Enhance the flavor of water by adding slices of fruits (like lemon, cucumber, or berries) and herbs (such as mint). It's a refreshing and natural option.

4. Sparkling Water:

- Why: Choose plain or flavored sparkling water without added sugars for a fizzy and enjoyable alternative to soda.

5. Green Tea:

- Why: Green tea is rich in antioxidants and offers a mild caffeine boost. You may eat it hot or cold.

6. Coconut Water:

- Why: Natural coconut water is a hydrating option that provides electrolytes. Choose varieties without added sugars.

7. Freshly Squeezed Juice:

- Why: If you enjoy fruit juice, consider making it fresh at home to control sugar content. Dilute with water or mix with sparkling water to reduce sweetness.

8. Vegetable Juice:

- Why: Blend vegetables like kale, spinach, cucumber, and celery for a nutrient-packed drink without added sugars.

9. Iced Herbal Tea:

- Why: Brew herbal tea, let it cool, and serve over ice for a flavorful and refreshing iced beverage.

10. Low-Fat Milk or Plant-Based Milk:

- Why: These options provide calcium and vitamin D. Choose unsweetened varieties for a healthier choice.

11. Kombucha:

- Why: Kombucha is a fermented tea with potential probiotic benefits. Select varieties with minimal added sugars.

12. Diluted Fruit Juice:

- Why: If you enjoy fruit juice, dilute it with water to reduce the sugar concentration. Gradually decrease the ratio over time.

13. Cold Brew Coffee:

- Why: If you like coffee, cold brew is a smoother and naturally sweeter option. Limit added sugars and high-calorie creamers.

14. Homemade Smoothies:

- Why: Blend fresh or frozen fruits with yogurt or plant-based milk. Avoid adding additional sweeteners for a naturally sweet treat.

15. Lemon Water:

- Why: Squeeze fresh lemon into water for a citrusy flavor without added sugars. Lemon water can also aid digestion.

16. Unsweetened Almond Milk:

- Why: Almond milk is a low-calorie and dairy-free alternative. Pick kinds without added sugars if you want to avoid them.

17. Cucumber Mint Refresher:

- Why: Combine cucumber slices and fresh mint in water for a cooling and flavorful drink.

Making these swaps gradually can help you transition away from sugary beverages while still enjoying tasty and healthful options. Remember to be mindful of portion sizes and read labels to avoid hidden sugars.

Overcoming Challenges in the Sugar-detox Journey

Embarking on a sugar detox journey can pose challenges, but overcoming them is key to success. Here are strategies to address common obstacles:

1. Sugar Cravings:

- Strategy: Gradually reduce sugar intake rather than going cold turkey. Select natural sweeteners sparingly, such as honey or maple syrup. When you're desiring something sweet, go for entire fruits.

2. Withdrawal Symptoms:

- Strategy: Stay hydrated, prioritize nutrient-rich foods, and incorporate regular meals. Gradually reducing caffeine can also help manage withdrawal symptoms.

3. Emotional Eating:

- Strategy: Identify emotional triggers for eating and find alternative coping

mechanisms, such as practicing
mindfulness, going for a walk, or
engaging in a hobby.

**4. Social Pressures:

- Strategy: Communicate your goals to
  friends and family, so they can support
  your choices. Bring your own sugar-free
  snacks to social events, and focus on
  the social aspect rather than the food.

**5. Hidden Sugars:

- Strategy: Read food labels carefully.
  Sugar hides under various names,
  including sucrose, high fructose corn
  syrup, and agave nectar. Choose whole,
  unprocessed foods to minimize hidden
  sugars.

6. Meal Planning:

- Strategy: Plan meals and snacks in advance to avoid impulsive food choices. Ensure balanced meals with a mix of proteins, healthy fats, and complex carbohydrates to keep you satisfied.

7. Craving Alternatives:

- Strategy: Find healthier alternatives to your favorite sugary treats. For example, replace candies with fruit, or opt for dark chocolate with a higher cocoa content.

8. Limited Food Options:

- Strategy: Explore a variety of nutrient-dense foods to keep your meals interesting. Try out various dishes and cuisines to find new favorites.

9. Mindful Eating:

- Strategy: Practice mindful eating by savoring each bite, paying attention to hunger and fullness cues, and enjoying the flavors and textures of your food.

10. Sugar in Beverages:

- Strategy: Replace sugary drinks with water, herbal tea, or sparkling water. Gradually reduce the amount of sugar or sweeteners you add to your coffee or tea.

11. **Education and Awareness:

- Strategy: Educate yourself about the impact of sugar on health. Understanding the benefits of reducing sugar can reinforce your commitment to the detox journey.

12. **Accountability:

- Strategy: Share your goals with a friend, family member, or a support group. Having someone to hold you accountable can be motivating and provide encouragement.

13. **Patience and Persistence:

- Strategy: Recognize that the sugar detox process takes time. Be patient with yourself, celebrate small victories, and focus on the long-term benefits of a reduced sugar lifestyle.

Remember that everyone's journey is unique, and it's okay to encounter challenges. Developing a positive mindset, seeking support, and making gradual changes can contribute to a successful sugar detox journey.

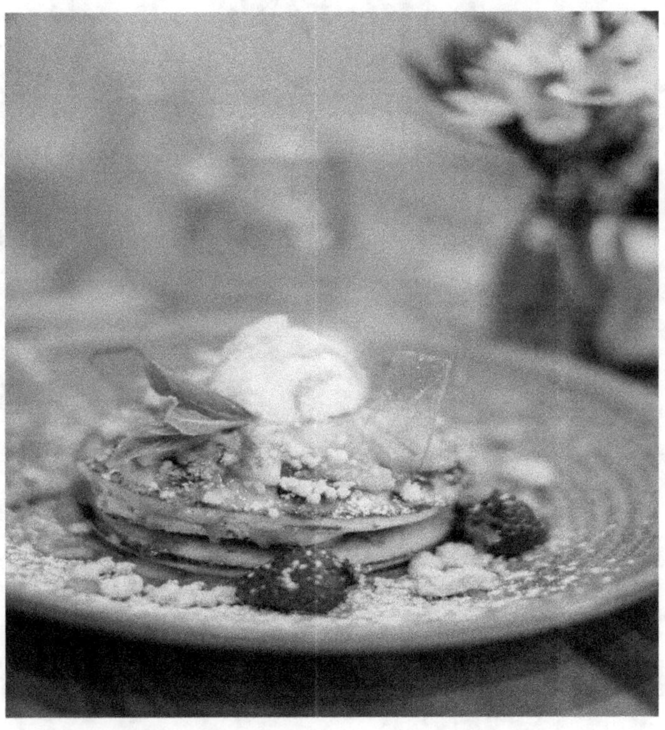

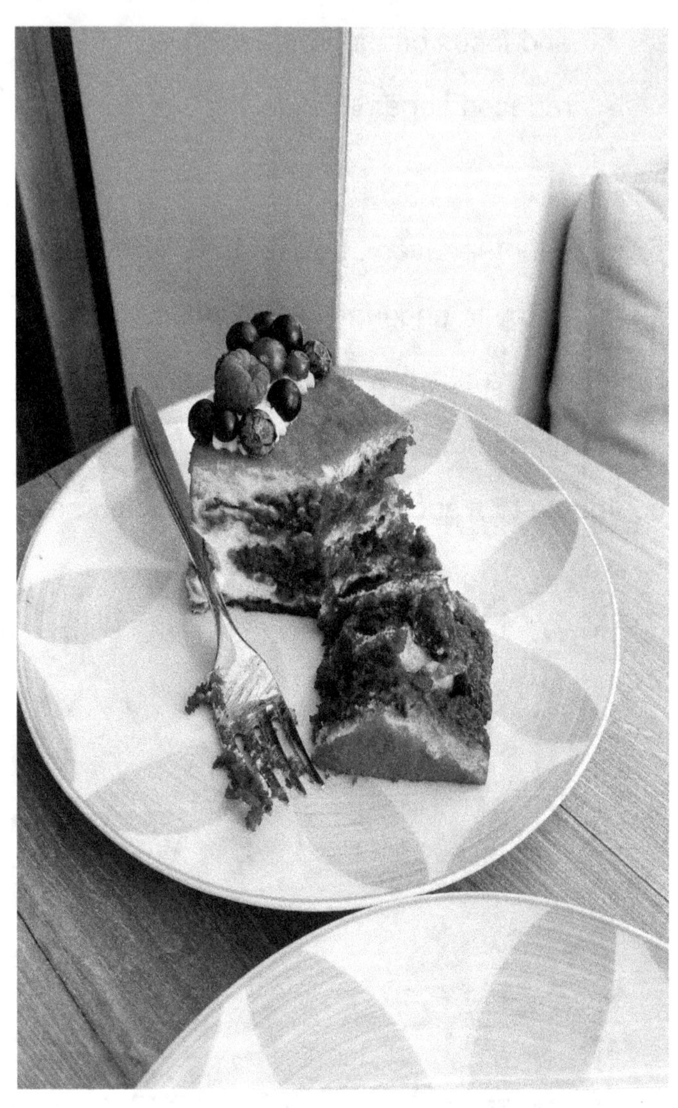

Chapter eight

Societal pressure and coping strategies

Societal pressure, especially related to dietary choices and lifestyle, can present challenges. Here are coping strategies to navigate societal pressure while maintaining your health goals:

**1. Communicate Your Choices:

- Coping Strategy: Clearly communicate your dietary choices to friends, family, and colleagues. Explain the reasons behind your decisions, fostering understanding and support.

2. Set Boundaries:

- Coping Strategy: Establish boundaries around discussions about food and health. Politely but firmly decline unwanted advice or criticism. Focus on your own well-being.

3. Educate Others:

- Coping Strategy: Share information about the benefits of your chosen lifestyle. Providing facts may dispel misconceptions and reduce pressure from others.

4. Lead by Example:

- Coping Strategy: Demonstrate the positive effects of your lifestyle through your own well-being. Leading by example can inspire others without engaging in confrontations.

**5. Find Like-Minded Communities:

- Coping Strategy: Seek out communities or groups that share similar health goals. Connecting with like-minded individuals can provide support and understanding.

**6. Confidence in Choices:

- Coping Strategy: Cultivate confidence in your decisions. Trusting your choices can help you navigate societal pressure with a sense of assurance.

7. Selective Sharing:

- Coping Strategy: Choose when and with whom to share details about your dietary choices. Not every situation may warrant a detailed explanation.

8. Celebrate Diversity:

- Coping Strategy: Embrace and celebrate diverse dietary preferences and choices. Encourage an inclusive environment where different perspectives are respected.

9. Mindful Responses:

- Coping Strategy: Respond mindfully to comments or questions. Choose to express gratitude for concern while

maintaining your commitment to your
health choices.

10. Be Open to Compromise:

- Coping Strategy: While maintaining your
core principles, be open to compromise
in certain social situations. Finding a
balance can reduce feelings of isolation.

11. Focus on Overall Well-being:

- Coping Strategy: Emphasize the holistic
benefits of your chosen lifestyle. Shift
the focus from appearance to overall
well-being, including mental health and
energy levels.

12. Seek Professional Guidance:

- Coping Strategy: Consult with
  healthcare professionals or nutritionists
  to solidify your health choices. Having
  expert guidance can boost your
  confidence in your decisions.

13. Respect for Others:

- Coping Strategy: Show respect for other
  people's choices, even if they differ from
  yours. A non-judgmental attitude can
  foster positive relationships.

14. Practice Assertiveness:

- Coping Strategy: Develop assertiveness
  skills to express your needs and choices
  confidently without being
  confrontational. This can help establish
  clear boundaries.

15. **Self-Reflection:

- Coping Strategy: Reflect on your own motivations and values regularly. Understanding why you make certain choices can reinforce your commitment and resilience.

Coping with societal pressure involves a combination of communication, confidence, and understanding. Remember that your health journey is personal, and finding a balance that works for you is crucial.

Reflection on Sugar-detox process

Reflecting on the sugar detox process is valuable for understanding your journey, acknowledging achievements, and identifying areas for continued improvement. Here are key aspects to consider:

**1. Initial Motivation:

- Reflect on what initially motivated you to undergo a sugar detox. This could be health concerns, energy levels, or a desire for overall well-being.

**2. Challenges Faced:

- Identify the challenges you encountered during the sugar detox. Whether it was cravings, social pressures, or emotional aspects, recognizing challenges is a crucial part of the reflection process.

**3. Successes and Achievements:

- Celebrate your successes, no matter
  how small. Recognize milestones such
  as reduced sugar intake, improved
  energy levels, or better overall health.

**4. Learnings and Insights:

- Consider what you've learned about
  yourself and your relationship with
  sugar. Recognize patterns, triggers, and
  the impact of dietary choices on your
  physical and mental well-being.

**5. Adaptation and Flexibility:

- Reflect on how well you adapted to the
  changes. Did you find alternatives to
  sugary snacks and beverages? Were
  you able to modify recipes or discover
  new, sugar-free favorites?

**6. Mindful Eating Habits:

- Assess how mindful you became about your eating habits. Did you develop a greater awareness of portion sizes, hunger cues, and the nutritional content of foods?

**7. Emotional Well-being:

- Explore the connection between your sugar intake and emotional well-being. Did you notice changes in mood, stress levels, or overall mental health during the detox?

**8. Social Interactions:

- Consider how social interactions influenced your sugar detox journey. Did you face challenges during gatherings

or find supportive environments among
friends and family?

9. Physical Changes:

- Reflect on any physical changes you
  observed. This could include changes in
  weight, skin health, energy levels, or
  improvements in sleep patterns.

10. Reintroduction of Natural Sugars:

- If applicable, consider how you
  reintroduced natural sugars from fruits
  back into your diet. How did your body
  respond, and did you notice any
  differences?

11. Future Goals:

- Define your future goals related to sugar intake. Are there specific habits you want to maintain or adjust? Consider setting realistic and sustainable goals for ongoing well-being.

**12. Self-Compassion:

- Be kind to yourself during the reflection process. Recognize that the sugar detox journey is a continuous process, and setbacks are opportunities for learning and growth.

**13. Support Systems:

- Evaluate the support systems you had in place. Reflect on how friends, family, or online communities contributed to or impacted your sugar detox journey.

**14. Celebrating Balance:

- Reflect on finding a balance that works for you. A sugar detox is not about complete elimination but about creating a sustainable and healthful relationship with sugar.

**15. Gratitude:

- Express gratitude for the effort and commitment you put into the sugar detox process. Acknowledge the positive steps you took towards prioritizing your health.

Reflection is a powerful tool for personal growth and continued well-being. Use your insights to inform future choices and maintain a healthful and balanced lifestyle.

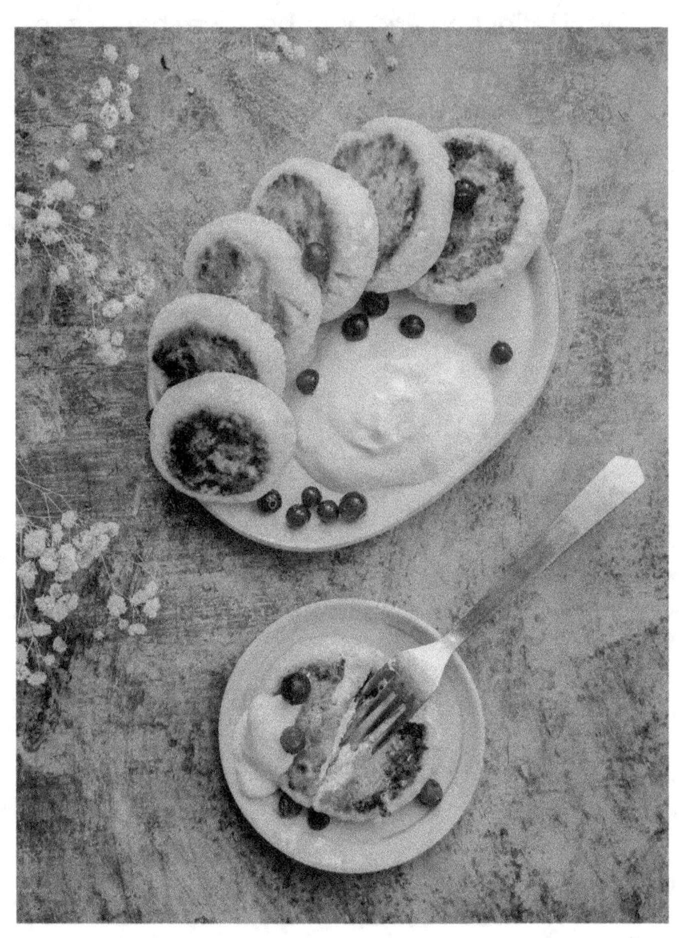

Conclusion

Embarking on a sugar detox journey as a beginner involves navigating various challenges and celebrating numerous victories. The initial motivation, whether rooted in health concerns, increased energy, or overall well-being, sets the tone for the entire process. Throughout the detox, individuals encounter challenges such as cravings, societal pressures, and emotional ties to food.

However, by employing strategies like mindful eating, setting boundaries, and finding alternatives, beginners can overcome these challenges. Successes in reducing sugar intake, adapting to healthier alternatives, and developing mindful eating habits should be acknowledged and celebrated. The sugar detox process extends beyond dietary changes, influencing emotional well-being, social interactions, and overall lifestyle.

Reflection plays a pivotal role in understanding personal motivations, learning about individual triggers, and recognizing the impact of sugar on both physical and mental health. As beginners navigate this journey, flexibility and adaptation to new habits become essential, with the ultimate goal of finding a sustainable and healthful balance.

Future goals may involve setting realistic intentions for ongoing well-being, reintroducing natural sugars mindfully, and maintaining support systems. It's crucial to approach the sugar detox journey with self-compassion, recognizing that setbacks are part of the learning process.

In conclusion, the sugar detox journey for beginners is a transformative process that goes beyond eliminating sugar from one's diet. It's about fostering a mindful and balanced relationship with food, understanding the emotional and societal aspects involved, and celebrating the continuous efforts towards a healthier lifestyle.